It's Always the Heart

Bible Study Guide

Arthur E. Constantine, MD

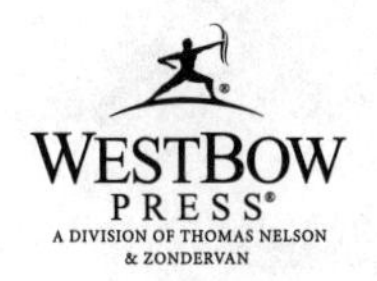

WestBow Press books may be ordered through booksellers or by contacting:

WestBow Press
A Division of Thomas Nelson & Zondervan
1663 Liberty Drive
Bloomington, IN 47403
www.westbowpress.com
1 (866) 928-1240

ISBN: 978-1-4908-7383-1 (sc)
ISBN: 978-1-4908-7382-4 (e)

Library of Congress Control Number: 2015907721

Printed in Ashland, Ohio

WestBow Press rev. date: 10/19/2015

Contents

STUDY GUIDE

Small Group Participant Worksheet

Chapter 1

A Haughty Heart

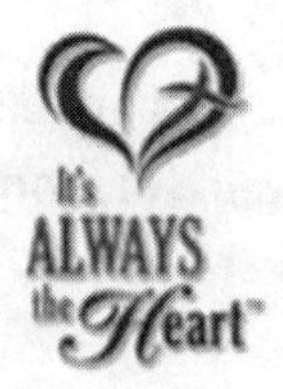

Before destruction a man's heart is haughty, but humility comes before honor.

Proverbs 18:12(ESV)

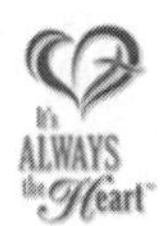

1. Preparation:

- Pray that God will use this message to strengthen the physical and spiritual hearts of you and all members in your group.
- Assign each meeting's opening prayer to a different group member.
- Read Chapter 1: A Haughty Heart and become familiar with the scripture references in the chapter.
- Share your thoughts and reflections on the worksheet.
- Be sensitive to the fact that diet and exercise-related topics may sometimes cause personal embarrassment – particularly if a group member struggles with his/her diet and/or exercise commitment to the group. The group should maintain an "encouragement-only" environment regardless of a member's progress or lack thereof.
- Remember: the primary goal of each chapter is to illustrate and emphasize the importance of God's design of the inseparability of the physical and spiritual heart. Keep the discussion focused on the chapter's goal.
- Try to adhere to the time recommendations for each topic of group discussion.

2. Thoughts: (25-30 Minutes)

A) Mr. Important is described early in the chapter as one who appears to be suffering from an overwhelming case of narcissism as defined by his attitude of self-importance, need for admiration and lack of empathy for anyone else. What does the Apostle Paul say about those who are "haughty" and "lovers of self"?

2 Timothy 3:1-4 (NKJV) But know this, that in the last days perilous times will come: For men will be lovers of themselves, lovers of money, boasters, proud, blasphemers, disobedient to parents, unthankful, unholy, unloving, unforgiving, slanderers, without self-control, brutal, despisers of good, traitors, headstrong, haughty, lovers of pleasure rather than lovers of God,

- Discuss the similarities between the type of behavior Paul references in 2 Timothy and Mr. Important's behavior with Dr. Constantine.

B) Stop for a moment and reflect on the number of people you encounter in your family, your workplace or your circle of friends who live their lives with an attitude of "self-love" similar to Mr. Important. How would you characterize their physical health?

What about their relationship with their family, friends and co-workers? Can you identify the link between their physical heart and their spiritual heart? How does this "self-love" heart issue apply to you?

- As the group members' observations and comments will likely gravitate toward how frequently we all encounter self-important friends, family and/or co-workers- try to focus the discussion on their observations of a self-important person (can use yourself) who suffers from spiritual heart problems and how it affects the person's physical heart. Refer to Mr. Important's spiritual emptiness and its effect on his physical heart.

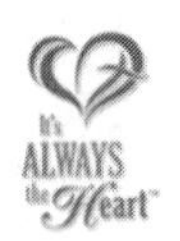

C) Aren't we all occasionally guilty of over-emphasizing the "importance" of our jobs, our priorities, our appearance, our family, etc.? How does this apply to you? If so, how do we prevent self-indulgence from recurring?

- Overcoming self-importance and selfishness has sometimes been called everyman's everyday curse. According to the Apostle Paul we must all deal with the "everyday curse" by dying unto ourselves everyday - by attempting to put others first …and ourselves last. *1 Corinthians 15:31 (NKJV) I affirm, by the boasting in you which I have in Christ Jesus our Lord, I die daily.*

D) Considering the sobering statistic that heart disease is the number one killer of men and women in this country, why do so many of us choose to ignore the facts that smoking, overeating, and lack of exercise – as well as other lifestyle-related issues – are among the leading causes of heart disease?

It is possible the group will become a bit uncomfortable at the introduction of this topic. Everyone attempts to rationalize their sins and shortcomings – particularly as it relates to overeating and lack of exercise. As a conversation starter, the following excerpt from a popular Bible commentary may be helpful in setting the stage for meaningful discussion of this sensitive topic:

- In *The Cost of Discipleship,* Dietrich Bonhoeffer penned the words, "Cheap grace is grace without discipleship, grace without the cross, grace without Jesus Christ, living and incarnate". Cheap grace means living as though God ignores or condones our sins. But

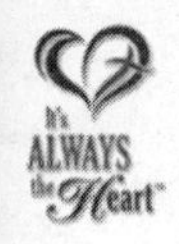

forgiveness means that sin is real, and must be dealt with. We cannot ignore it, because God does not ignore it. The denial of sin is not grace: it is a lie. Cheap grace means living without the demand of obedience upon us. *1 John 2: IVP New Testament Commentaries*

- What has led us to believe that God condones us eating unhealthy fast foods…a fast-paced lifestyle?

- What has led us to believe that God condones our unwillingness to exercise and maintain our wonderfully made bodies?

- What does God say about the daily *exercise* of our spiritual heart?

3. Personal Reflections: (25-30 minutes)

A) Do I honestly consider exercise as a time of fellowship with God or simply a chore that I do begrudgingly for the sake of my vanity and pride? Or, do I exercise for enjoyment, stress relief and life-changing benefits? Elaborate on this reflection.

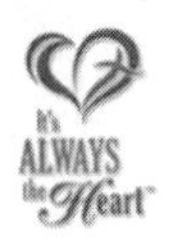

- According to Gym, Health & Fitness Industry research (from 2011), "Gym membership numbers have increased considerably over the past 10 years rising from 36.3 million to 42.8 million members who – on average – find themselves in a gym a couple of days a week."... are these fitness-minded millions joining in record numbers to honor God, or help themselves feel better, live longer and healthier while honoring God with the effort?

- If you decided to approach an exercise regimen as a special time to fellowship with God…do you think it would make a difference in your being successful in achieving a healthy heart and body? Why or why not?

B) Am I willing to commit to God, myself and the group to even a modest daily regimen of heart-healthy exercise? How will I make this commitment? (Consult recommended exercise routines/regimens if just getting started)

(It is important to remind everyone that the commitment to a daily regimen of exercise should be preceded by a clearance from their personal physician. Further, group members need to understand that the regimen/routine will vary greatly between each member due to a number of factors – including but not limited to – age, height & weight, pre-existing conditions and general condition of overall health and current exercise conditioning.)

- Encourage group members to exercise together (e.g. the "accountability partner" approach) if possible. How might this help?

- Explain that during each group meeting, each member will be encouraged to discuss their previous week's progress or lack thereof. How might this help?

C) Do my eating habits reflect a God-centered approach to life, work and family - or are they, like Mr. Important, simply an example of self-indulgence that I choose to rationalize because of my lifestyle?

- Recent government studies have estimated the percentage of overweight adults in the U.S at a staggering 60%-68% (overweight children represent an alarming 33%). Citizens at or near the poverty level are often excused due to not having enough money to buy anything other than high-calorie, high-fat content foods (Even though economists have repeatedly proven that a family's food dollar is stretched significantly when their food needs are purchased at a grocery store – versus high-priced, fast food). For nearly everyone else, however, there doesn't appear to be a reasonable excuse. Is it simply their love of food, the wrong kind of food, their lack of self-control or, as Paul suggests, a deep self-centeredness where their appetites and desires come first as in *Philippians 3:19* where he states "*...their god is their stomach...*"?

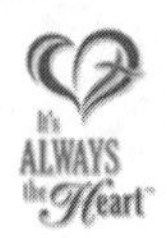

D) Am I willing to commit to God, myself and the group to make a concerted effort to change my eating habits to include a more nutritionally balanced diet of heart-healthy foods? How do I plan to make this commitment? (See recommended diet/ nutrition guide or utilize outside source)

- Although this question may lead to some members to express a heartfelt desire to change their eating habits – they may not have the motivation to follow through. Thus, it is important, that each group member be encouraged to assist struggling members in their commitment to take control of their weight. Prayer, meal planning assistance and phone calls of encouragement will all be welcomed to those in the fellowship who need help.

E) Is my heart a humble one, defined by who I am in Christ – or a self-important one defined by how successful I am in the world? Elaborate.

At first glance, this question may seem easy to answer. Surely everyone wants to think of themselves as having a humble heart. However, if the participant is being honest with him/herself, it will likely generate a significant amount of self-effacing discussion.

F) Am I willing to commit to God, myself and the group to the daily spiritual exercise of my heart through the study of God's Word? How do I plan to implement this commitment?

What is God revealing specifically to my heart through the story of Mr. Important and how will it impact my physical and spiritual heart health?

Chapter 1 Scripture Re-cap:
Proverbs 18:12
Psalm 101:5
Proverbs 16:5
Proverbs 8:17
Colossians 3:17

Encourage group members to read and meditate on the scriptures referenced in each chapter.

Closing Prayer

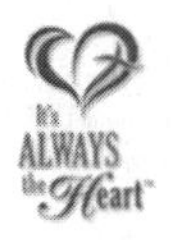

NOTES

Chapter 2

A Joyful Heart

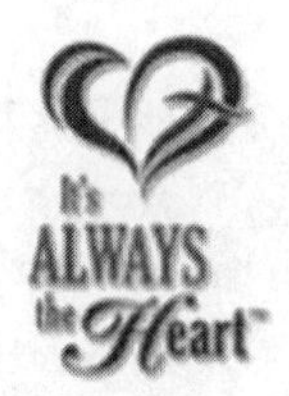

A cheerful heart is good medicine, but a crushed spirit dries up the bones.

Proverbs 17:22

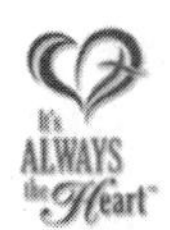

1. <u>Preparation:</u>

- Pray that God will use this message to strengthen the physical and spiritual hearts of you and all members in your group.
- Assign each meeting's opening prayer to a different group member.
- Read Chapter 2: A Joyful Heart and become familiar with the scripture references in the chapter.
- Share your thoughts and reflections on the worksheet.
- Be sensitive to the fact that diet and exercise-related topics may sometimes cause personal embarrassment – particularly if a group member struggles with his/her diet and/or exercise commitment to the group. The group should maintain an "encouragement-only" environment regardless of a member's progress or lack thereof.
- Remember: the primary goal of each chapter is to illustrate and emphasize the importance of God's design of the inseparability of the physical and spiritual heart. Keep the discussion focused on the chapter's goal.
- Try to adhere to the time recommendations for each topic of group discussion.

2. <u>Thoughts: (25-30 Minutes)</u>

A) It might have seemed unfair to read about an energetic, healthy woman like Mary Tallent having to endure the pain and trauma of a heart attack. After all, she was dedicated to exercise, good nutrition, and living a Christ-filled life. Yet, she found herself in an emergency helicopter ride to a hospital cardiac cath lab to save her life. What lesson is God trying to teach us when we experience or read about similar situations of "bad things

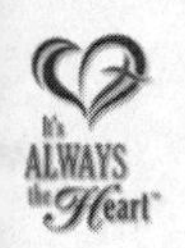

happening to good people?" What do the scriptures have to say on this subject?

- *1 Peter 2: 19-21 For it is commendable if a man bears up under the pain of unjust suffering because he is conscious of God. But how is it to your credit if you receive a beating for doing wrong and endure it? But if you suffer for doing good and you endure it, this is commendable before God. To this you were called, because Christ suffered for you, leaving you an example, that you should follow in his steps.*

- *Romans 8:35 Who shall separate us from the love of Christ? Shall trouble or hardship or persecution or famine or nakedness or danger or sword?*

- Discuss the importance of remembering as Christians, through any trial, God is always in control and that we are never separated from Him. Whatever pain He allows, He will heal.

B) Dr. Constantine points out that "God never promised us a life free of health problems…rather, he promised to never leave us regardless of the obstacles" we face. Does that mean that our pursuit of a healthy physical and spiritual heart may be in vain?

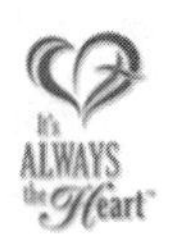

- Consider resolving the thought behind this question by steering the group's discussion toward the eternal truth that nothing done for the Lord is done in vain: *John 16:33 I have told you these things, so that in me you may have peace. In this world you will have trouble. But take heart! I have overcome the world.*

C) If Mary Tallent was indeed one of God's special servants in which"...people saw God's light through her life and wanted what she had," why would God allow such a precious witness's life to come so perilously close to death?

- As additional follow-up to Thought "C", here is another potential discussion point: As difficult as it is to comprehend, we live in a flawed and fallen world wherein trial and tribulation are to not only be expected but praised. *2 Corinthians 12: 9-10 But he said to me, "My grace is sufficient for you, for my power is made perfect in weakness." Therefore I will boast all the more gladly about my weaknesses, so that Christ's power may rest on me. That is why, for Christ's sake, I delight in weaknesses, in insults, in hardships, in persecutions, in difficulties. For when I am weak, then I am strong.*

- Like Mary Tallent, who do we find in our community – or in the news - that may be considered someone whose enduring of hardships and persecutions present a strong praiseworthy witness for Christ? (the answers to this could range from missionaries, to pro athletes,

to everyday acquaintances who live a life of strong witness...each worthy of discussion.) *1 Peter 1:6-7 In this you greatly rejoice, though now for a little while you may have had to suffer grief in all kinds of trials. These have come so that your faith—of greater worth than gold, which perishes even though refined by fire—may be proved genuine and may result in praise, glory and honor when Jesus Christ is revealed.*

- Satan was introduced in Genesis and we were warned by God to avoid his devouring our lives, *1Peter 5:8 Be self-controlled and alert. Your enemy the devil prowls around like a roaring lion looking for someone to devour.* Open a discussion about how Satan can use illness and disease as a wound in which he can prey upon.

3. <u>Personal Reflections: (25-30 minutes)</u>

A) If I strive to develop and healthy physical and spiritual heart, could I end up like Mary Tallent? Does that mean I will always walk around in fear – even if I do my best at maintaining good health? Or, does this give me a stronger foundation to handle adversity when it comes my way? Elaborate on this reflection.

- There are numerous times in scripture where we are reassured that we do not have to be afraid: *1 Peter 3:14 But even if you should suffer for what is right, you are blessed. "Do not fear what they fear; do not be frightened."*

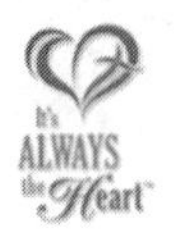

- For added perspective, it may be good to ask the group to compare the difference in how their faith helps them deal with fear of known/predictable trials in comparison to unknown/unexpected ones.

- Consider punctuating the "fear factor" discussion with God's glorious promise found in *James 1:12 Blessed is the man who perseveres under trial, because when he has stood the test, he will receive the crown of life that God has promised to those who love him*

B) Can I honestly say that I will strive to improve my heart health because I want to, first, honor God…or am I doing it for some other reason?

- To approach this topic, it may be helpful, as well as an interesting and insightful exercise in personal motivation, to have each member of the group make two columns from a blank sheet of paper. On one column, have them write "RIGHT REASONS"…and in the other column have them write "WRONG REASONS". Then after everyone has made an attempt to list their reasons – as suggested in the "B" question above – discuss some or all of them. Inevitably, "fear" is going to enter into the discussion and draw a corollary to the "A" reflection previously discussed.

- *1 Thessalonians 2:4* is an appropriate scripture to help draw this discussion point to a scriptural close...*On the contrary, we speak as men approved by God to be entrusted with the gospel. We are not trying to please men but God, who tests our hearts.*

C) Why, like Mary Tallent, do I allow self-pity and doubt to creep into my thoughts when faced with illness, discouraging me about that which I know is true regarding my health, life, and God's Word?

- A good point of entry for this topic is to engage the group in a comparative discussion of the Apostle Paul – and the extreme hardships he endured during the days of the early church *(2 Corinthians 11:23-28)* – as they relate to the modern (and comparatively mundane) moments of discouragement that many Christians consider themselves "burdened" with today.

- Additional scripture appropriate to this topic is *Galatians 6:9 Let us not become weary in doing good, for at the proper time we will reap a harvest if we do not give up.*

D) Do I truly believe that everything that happens in my life - good and bad – happens in the context of God's perfect plan and deserves to be praised...or, do I allow myself to become discouraged into believing the bad times are a result of my failures?

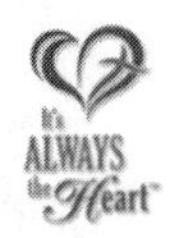

- It is often said that for us mere mortal men and women, success is not final, nor is failure fatal! They are simply a part of God's plan for our lives.

- Thus, we all need to be reminded that just as Christ's death was in God's perfect plan, we cannot allow ourselves to become discouraged in the darkness of past failures.

How is God asking my heart to be joyful in this season of my life through the story of Mary Tallent?

Chapter 2 Scripture Recap:
Proverbs 17:22
Romans 8:17
Psalm 23:4
1 Chronicles 16:11
1 Thessalonians 5:16-18

Encourage group members to read and meditate on the scriptures referenced in each chapter.

Closing Prayer

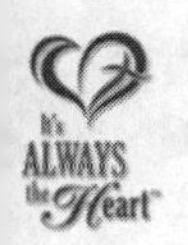

NOTES

Chapter 3

Addiction

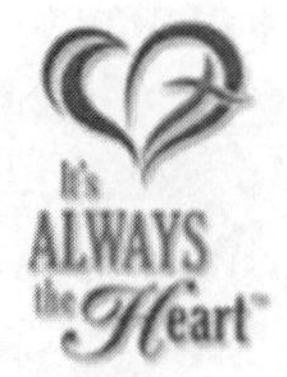

For the grace of God that brings salvation has appeared to all men. It teaches us to say "No" to ungodliness and worldly passions, and to live self-controlled, upright and godly lives in this present age, while we wait for the blessed hope—the glorious appearing of our great God and Savior, Jesus Christ, who gave himself for us to redeem us from all wickedness and to purify for himself a people that are his very own, eager to do what is good.

Titus 2: 11-14

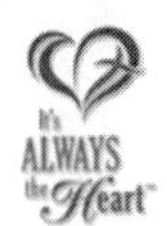

1. Preparation:

- Pray that God will use this message to strengthen the physical and spiritual hearts of you and all members in your group.
- Assign each meeting's opening prayer to a different group member.
- Read Chapter 3: Addiction and become familiar with the scripture references in the chapter.
- Share your thoughts and reflections on the worksheet.
- Be sensitive to the fact that diet, exercise, and topics related to personal shortcomings/weaknesses may sometimes cause personal embarrassment – particularly if a group member struggles with his/her diet and/or exercise commitment to the group. The group should maintain an "encouragement-only" environment regardless of a member's progress or lack thereof.
- Remember: the primary goal of each chapter is to illustrate and emphasize the importance of God's design of the inseparability of the physical and spiritual heart. Keep the discussion focused on the chapter's goal.
- Try to adhere to the time recommendations for each topic of group discussion.

2. Thoughts: (25-30 Minutes)

A) The two Jacobs illustrated in this chapter, admittedly, may not be the typical people we know and interact with on a daily basis (as far as we know), yet we all have weaknesses that might be considered addictions. Carefully scrutinize your addictions. What does God say about our weaknesses/addictions?

- Since people often feel frightened and defeated when discussing the topic of addiction, it is good to have the

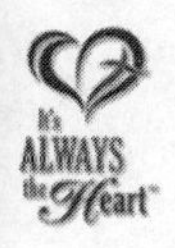

beginning of the conversation rooted in the hope of scripture as illustrated in *1 Corinthians 10:13 (TNIV) No temptation has overtaken you except what is common to us all. And God is faithful; he will not let you be tempted beyond what you can bear. But when you are tempted, he will also provide a way out so that you can endure it.*

- Next, in an attempt to keep the group from too narrowly or classically defining the term "addiction", guide the group conversation toward its broader identification by referencing Webster's medical definition: *Addiction - the persistent compulsive use of a substance known by the user to be physically, psychologically, or socially harmful.* Ask for the group to declare that which they feel are addictions that plague people from all walks of life; personally (on paper or verbally) disclose those addictions that plague you.

- To resolve this Thought, reference *2 Corinthians 7:1* as God's instruction on why it is important to rid ourselves of addictions…*Since we have these promises, dear friends, let us purify ourselves from everything that contaminates body and spirit, perfecting holiness out of reverence for God.*

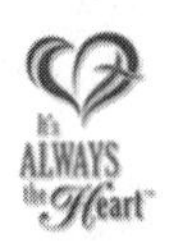

B) How many people do we see at home, work, school or play that seemingly "have it all together", yet when things are revealed – as all things are always seen by God – all of them are burdened with some kind of addiction? What are the addictions you observe them struggling with and what impact do the addictions have on their lives? Search your own heart and try to bring to light the addictions with which you struggle and what impact they have on your life.

- More significant than the list of addictions likely discussed by the group here, it is also important to help the group consider how the addictions consume our heart and interfere with our life, as opposed to the perceived severity or degree of sinfulness an addiction may have. Think of addictions that have a grip on you personally or addictions in general. Are there levels of interference caused by the addictions in our lives that:
    - slightly distract us from God's purpose in our lives.
    - consume and distract us from God's purpose in our lives.
    - consume and interfere with all the blessings God has for our lives yet are not obstacles to life everlasting.
    - disqualify us from life everlasting.
    - Can the same addiction have a different result on the life and/or salvation of different individuals? How can this be true?

- Scripture suggestion: *1 Corinthians 4:5 Therefore judge nothing before the appointed time; wait till the Lord comes. He will bring to light what is hidden in darkness*

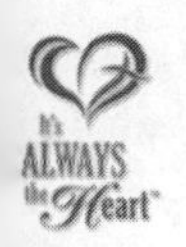

and will expose the motives of mens hearts. At that time each will receive his praise from God.

C) The name "Jacob" in the book of Genesis in the Old Testament – "the deceiver" – is defined in Webster's dictionary as…*one who makes believe that which is not true; tricks or misleads.* How then are we all deceivers when it comes to the addictions we face? How do we see our addictions in comparison to the two Jacobs in the chapter or even to others we know? How do you think God sees our addictions by comparison?

- It is possible that some in the group will become a bit uncomfortable at the introduction of this topic. Everyone attempts to rationalize their sins and shortcomings – and even addictions – so proceed gently and with caution.

- Use the following scripture as a reference point of hope in the face of seemingly hopeless situations surrounding addictive temptations: *Hebrews 4:15-16 For we do not have a high priest who is unable to empathize with our weaknesses, but we have one who has been tempted in every way, just as we are—yet he did not sin. Let us then approach God's throne of grace with confidence, so that we may receive mercy and find grace to help us in our time of need*

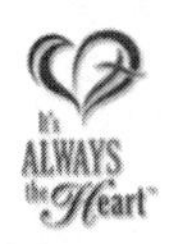

D) Considering many addictions (like smoking, over-eating and drugs, to name a few) affect our physical heart and body, why do so many of us – even those who have suffered a heart problem – continue with the addictions despite this knowledge?...or, address only some addictions while continuing with others? Do some of us follow nutritious, antioxidant diets and/or exercise daily in an attempt to mitigate the effect our ongoing addictions have on our health and life? Elaborate on how this applies to you.

- Discussion point: Addiction is often referred to as a disease of revolving denial and regret…denial of the problem and its tortuous grip on the addicted followed by regret of the denial. In short, the heart's denial of the addiction causes many people – even those who have suffered with a heart problem – to ignore treatment of their addiction.

3. <u>Personal Reflections: (25-30 minutes)</u>

A) Is my heart ready to 1) confess and admit my addictions by turning them over to Jesus Christ for strength in freeing me from the bondage of these addictions, or 2) confess and admit some of my addictions while holding on to others as I 'bargain' with God? Is my heart hardened to confessing any of my addictions despite the fact that doing so may interfere with the blessings God wants to pour into my life? Elaborate on how these questions apply to you personally.

- Encourage the group to outline the differences between a full measure of surrender versus a "strings attached" surrender of addictions.

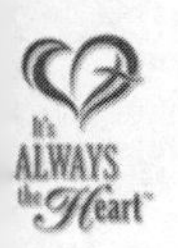

- Scripture support: *1 Peter 5:6-7 Humble yourselves, therefore, under God's mighty hand, that he may lift you up in due time. Cast all your anxiety on him because he cares for you.*

B) How are my addictions affecting my spiritual and physical heart health? How do I see myself and my addictions relative to others and their addictions? Can I live a normal life – and can I even get to Heaven – burdened with addictions?

- Discussion: Since we now know that the spiritual and physical hearts are inseparable, we must conclude that all addictions are damaging to both dimensions of the heart. Yet most of us suffering from addictions tend to deny the severity of our particular addiction whether it be drugs, alcohol, overeating or some other substance or dependency.

- Scriptural assurances of Heaven – even in light of burdensome addictions:

- *Colossians 2:13: When you were dead in your sins and in the uncircumcision of your sinful nature, God made you alive with Christ. He forgave us all our sins,*

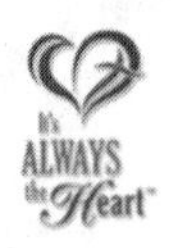

C) Am I willing to commit to God, myself and the group to take an honest inventory of the destructive addictions and habits in my life and devote the time for spiritual exercise of my heart through daily study of God's Word to help me rid my life of addictions so I become all God wants me to be? How do I envision this commitment taking shape in my life? How will this be an on-going battle?

- Unfortunately, people are often unwilling to surrendering to the reality of God's ever-present grace as illustrated in *2 Corinthians 12:9-10 But he said to me, "My grace is sufficient for you, for my power is made perfect in weakness." Therefore I will boast all the more gladly about my weaknesses, so that Christ's power may rest on me. That is why, for Christ's sake, I delight in weaknesses, in insults, in hardships, in persecutions, in difficulties. For when I am weak, then I am strong*

D) Am I willing to put negative addictions aside and replace them with physically uplifting "good habits" in order to receive the bounty God is waiting to give me? How will I make this "exchange" and how will I make it permanent?

- *1 John 5:3-4 (TNIV) In fact, this is love for God: to keep his commands. And his commands are not burdensome, for everyone born of God overcomes the world. This is the victory that has overcome the world, even our faith.*

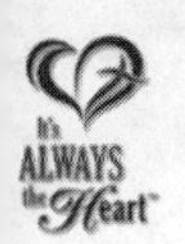

Ask for and discuss responses to the following two questions:

- What have you done up to now to successfully overcome some of your addictions?

- What are some of the recurring stumbling blocks to success?

How is God trying to break through to my heart and release the chains that inprison me with this chapter on addictions?

Chapter 3 Scripture Recap:
Titus 2: 11-14
1 Peter 5:8
1 Samuel 16:7
John 3:20
Proverbs 17:24
Jeremiah 29:11

Encourage group members to read and meditate on the scriptures referenced in each chapter.

Closing Prayer

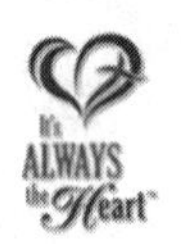

NOTES

STUDY GUIDE

Small Group Participant Worksheet

Chapter 4

Searching

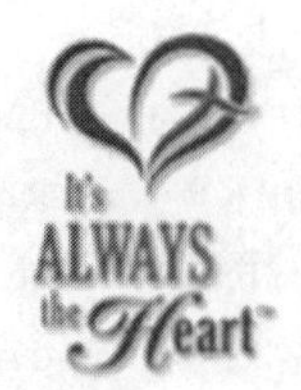

But seek his kingdom, and these things will be given to you as well.

Luke 12:31

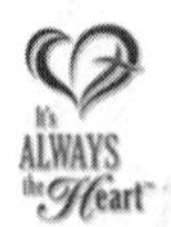

1. Preparation:

- Pray that God will use this message to strengthen the physical and spiritual hearts of you and all members in your group.
- Assign each meeting's opening prayer to a different group member.
- Read Chapter 4: Searching and become familiar with the scripture references in the chapter.
- Share your thoughts and reflections on the worksheet.
- Be sensitive to the fact that diet and exercise-related topics may sometimes cause personal embarrassment – particularly if a group member struggles with his/her diet and/or exercise commitment to the group. The group should maintain an "encouragement-only" environment regardless of a member's progress or lack thereof.
- Remember: the primary goal of each chapter is to illustrate and emphasize the importance of God's design of the inseparability of the physical and spiritual heart. Keep the discussion focused on the chapter's goal.
- Try to adhere to the time recommendations for each topic of group discussion.

2. Thoughts: (25-30 Minutes)

A) Much like Joanne in this chapter, many of us find ourselves searching for *things* in life that will give us peace. Without peace, nothing we do in life can settle our anxious hearts - even when we are where God wants us. What does God say about peace and how to find it?

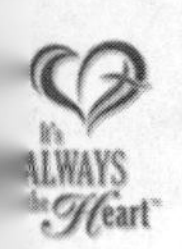

- First, the scripture is clear about the effect of anxiety on our hearts: *Proverbs 12:25 An anxious heart weighs a man down, but a kind word cheers him up.*

- Next, in order to fully grasp the issue of "finding" peace, it may be good to encourage the group to revisit that which the scriptures tell us is the reason that we do not experience peace. In Genesis we are reminded that mankind was created for fellowship with God. Thus, when we are separated from Him, we rob ourselves from the enjoyment of peace that comes from fellowship with Him. *John 14:27 Peace I leave with you; my peace I give you. I do not give to you as the world gives. Do not let your hearts be troubled and do not be afraid.*

B) Think for a moment about yourself and/or others around you – family, friends, acquaintances and co-workers who are always talking about themselves as it relates to 'what they are doing', constantly building themselves up, yet never seemingly content with that which they have and/or who they really are. Why is it difficult to develop a close relationship with them? What are the underlying issues that prevent us from developing close relationships with these individuals? How does the study of God's Word help us overcome this unrest and help put things in proper perspective?

- After discussing the difficulties of developing relationships with people who are self-absorbed, ask the group to identify that which lies at the core of an

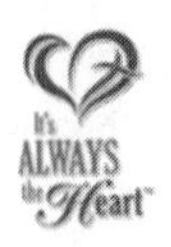

individual's behavior that prevents them from expressing genuine interest in the lives of others?....Selfish pride plays a major role and is addressed countless times in scripture. It is a spiritual weakness that can only be overcome by asking God for its removal: *Philippians 2:3-4 Do nothing out of selfish ambition or vain conceit, but in humility consider others better than yourselves. Each of you should look not only to your own interests, but also to the interests of others.*

- Ask what effect self-absorbed people have on their spiritual heart and the spiritual hearts of those they encounter: *1 Peter 5:5 ...All of you, clothe yourselves with humility toward one another, because, "God opposes the proud but gives grace to the humble."*

C) Admittedly, it is difficult to know the true path God has for our lives. How do we apply study of the Bible to our lives to help us know precisely where He wants us and, precisely where He wants us to go? Is it only after looking back that we see these things or is this something we can know while going through our life?

- This is often a perplexing issue and discussion. We all sometimes tend to wander and follow a trial-and-error approach in an attempt to discern the appointed path God has for our lives, yet it is clear that His Word is the primary tool we need to equip us for the journey. We would never think of playing tennis without a racket,

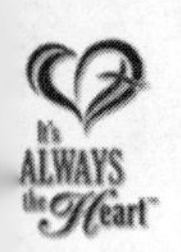

or repairing a car without the proper tools, or going on a cross-country trip without a map or a GPS system. So, it only makes sense that we carry God's Word with us on our life journey: *Psalm 119:105 Your word is a lamp to my feet and a light for my path.*

- Once we begin to understand God's will, commands, principles and impressions as we read them in His Holy Word, we can then begin charting a course for a life that is congruent with His perfect plan.

D) Joanne's circumstance was described as one of finally gaining the "freedom to find her purpose in corporate America". Yet she, like many of us, was disappointed once she reached the destination to which she had been searching. Why do you suppose this happens?

- Ask the group to share personal "be careful what you wish for" stories about how a long-anticipated journey to delight…turned quickly to despair. It is important here to emphasize that disappointment sometimes pushes us closer to our destiny and purpose even though our expectations were not what we thought they would (or should) be.

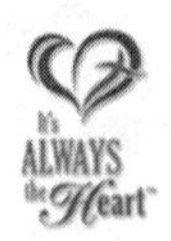

- Scripture support: *Proverbs 16:9 (TNIV) In their hearts human beings plan their course, but the LORD establishes their steps.*

3. Personal Reflections: (25-30 minutes)

A) It is well known that stress and worry can adversely affect our health – and I believe can even cause the cells our body to *cringe.* How does stress affect your life? Can we think and talk about a problem excessively to the point that we actually cause that which we worry about to become a reality? How might this happen?

- What can we do from the standpoint of diet and exercise to combat the effects of stress on our lives?

- What can we do from the standpoint of daily fellowship with God to alleviate the effects of stress on our lives?

- Ask the group to reveal ways in which they (or friends/family/etc.) attempt to combat and/or control stress. Does anyone answer with diet and exercise? If so, ask them to explain how diet and exercise helps them to mitigate stress. If not, use this moment to encourage those who have undertaken a diet and exercise regimen to take notice of any change in their stress levels as they

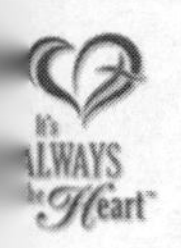

continue toward their goal of a healthier physical and spiritual heart.

- Suggested scripture for assurance that God is bigger than all of our worries, disappointments and problems:

- *Philippians 4:6-7 (TNIV) Do not be anxious about anything, but in every situation, by prayer and petition, with thanksgiving, present your requests to God. And the peace of God, which transcends all understanding, will guard your hearts and your minds in Christ Jesus.*

- *1 Peter 5:6-7 Humble yourselves, therefore, under God's mighty hand, that he may lift you up in due time. Cast all your anxiety on him because he cares for you.*

B) As was the case with Joanne's heart attack, do we truly feel as though God is with us in the midst of traumatic trials…or do we feel all alone? Elaborate on this reflection. Why do you think we have a tendency to forget God is with us during trying times?

- Personal trials – particularly those involving pain – tend to drive us to a point of believing that hope has vanished, leaving us to feel as though no one is with us – not even God. However, our attitude during trying times is often a statement of the strength of our faith.

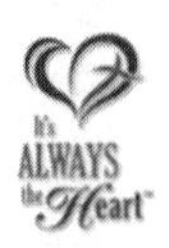

- Scripture support that underscores the fact that no matter what trials we face, all things are under the sovereign authority of Jesus Christ:

- *Isaiah 43:1-2 (TNIV) But now, this is what the LORD says—he who created you, Jacob, he who formed you, Israel: "Do not fear, for I have redeemed you; I have summoned you by name; you are mine. When you pass through the waters, I will be with you; and when you pass through the rivers, they will not sweep over you. When you walk through the fire, you will not be burned; the flames will not set you ablaze.*

C) What are the scriptures saying to me in *Colossians 3:15 "Let the peace of Christ rule in your hearts,..."*?

- How do you personalize this scripture to your own life? Would you be willing to share your *peace* with the group?

D) Looking at your life, how has God's hand been there all along, supporting and guiding your steps along life's path?

- Here are a few of the numerous scriptural references of how God guides our steps:

- *Proverbs 3:6 in all your ways acknowledge him, and he will make your paths straight.*

- *Psalm 119:105 Your word is a lamp to my feet and a light for my path (+ commentary: Apart from which I could only grope about in darkness)*

- *Proverbs 4:10-12 Listen, my son, accept what I say, and the years of your life will be many. I guide you in the way of wisdom and lead you along straight paths. When you walk, your steps will not be hampered; when you run, you will not stumble.*

How might God be trying to use this chapter on searching to help my heart find it's way?

Chapter 4 Scripture Re-cap:

Luke 12:31
Psalm 23:3
Philippians 4:11
1 Peter 3:11
Psalm 334:18
Hebrews 11:1
1 Thessalonians 5:17
John 16:33
Hebrews 13:5
Proverbs 27:19
Colossians 3:15
Matthew 6:33
Philippians 4:11-12
1 Corinthians 14:33
Joshua 1:7-8
Psalm 69:32

Encourage group members to read and meditate on the scriptures referenced in each chapter.

Closing Prayer

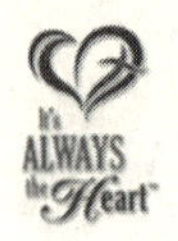

NOTES

STUDY GUIDE

Small Group Participant Worksheet

Chapter 5

Commitment

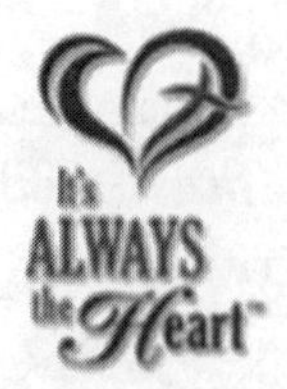

Commit your way to the Lord, Trust also in Him, And He shall bring it to pass.

Psalm 37:5 NKJV

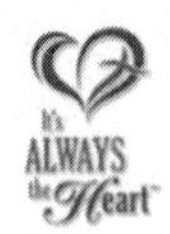

1. Preparation:

- Pray that God will use this message to strengthen the physical and spiritual hearts of you and all members in your group.
- Assign each meeting's opening prayer to a different group member.
- Read Chapter 5: Commitment and become familiar with the scripture references in the chapter.
- Share your thoughts and reflections on the worksheet.
- Be sensitive to the fact that diet and exercise-related topics may sometimes cause personal embarrassment – particularly if a group member struggles with his/her diet and/or exercise commitment to the group. The group should maintain an "encouragement-only" environment regardless of a member's progress or lack thereof.
- Remember: the primary goal of each chapter is to illustrate and emphasize the importance of God's design of the inseparability of the physical and spiritual heart. Keep the discussion focused on the chapter's goal.
- Try to adhere to the time recommendations for each topic of group discussion.

2. Thoughts: (25-30 Minutes)

A) Dr. Constantine characterized patient Jim Oliver as a kind of joy-filled person whose godly attitude represents "a true reflection of God's joy in their life." What does the Bible tell us lies at the core of living a joy-filled life? How does one go through myocardial infarction, coronary artery bypass surgery or internal cardiac defibrillator procedure, or any disease process for that matter, and still be joy-filled?

- The dictionary defines "joy" as *a deep feeling or condition of happiness or contentment.* Ask each member to give their personal explanation of "joy".

- Then ask each to consider that which lies at the very essence or core of a joy-filled life? Focus the discussion on the fact that true joy of comes from knowing we are blessed with an abundance of praiseworthy things in our lives: *Philippians 4:8 (TNIV) Finally, brothers and sisters, whatever is true, whatever is noble, whatever is right, whatever is pure, whatever is lovely, whatever is admirable—if anything is excellent or praiseworthy—think about such things..*

- As referenced in a previous chapter, the following passage from the book of James is a comforting scripture to reinforce our faith in the face of trials like the cardiac health issues asked in this question – *James 1:2-4 (TNIV) Consider it pure joy, my brothers and sisters, whenever you face trials of many kinds, because you know that the testing of your faith produces perseverance. Let perseverance finish its work so that you may be mature and complete, not lacking anything.*

B) What is your typical response to someone who asks you, "How are you doing today?" Do you always respond with a godly

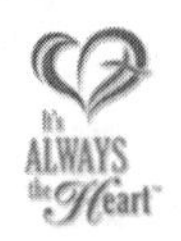

attitude, or do you allow daily distractions and doubtfulness steal the joy in your heart? How do we avoid the obstacles that rob us of having a joyful heart?

- Discuss the groups' various responses to the lead question. Then discuss the everyday life emotions and events that sometimes cause our hearts to not necessarily reflect a joy-filled, godly attitude – and how we can avoid them. Finally, introduce *John 10:10* as both and instruction and hope as it relates to our living a full and joy-filled life… *The thief comes only to steal and kill and destroy; I have come that they may have life, and have it to the full.*

- The ability to enjoy the life God has given us comes from Him – not ourselves and the things, activities, and pursuits that sometimes consume us. Further, we can help to avoid joy stealing distractions by understanding the importance of joy and enjoyment from a scriptural perspective – even in our toils; *Ecclesiastes 2:24 (NKJV) Nothing is better for a man than that he should eat and drink, and that his soul should enjoy good in his labor. This also, I saw, was from the hand of God.*

C) What does it mean when we "commit" to someone or something? How do we become Christ-like when we commit to the things that are beneficial to our health? How do we commit to a daily relationship with God?

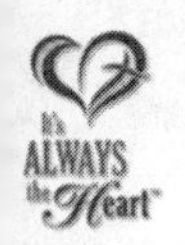

- Discuss the meaning of "commit" and its embodiment of a pledge, promise or obligation. Then ask the group to name instances of how we fail in our commitments to each other as Christian brothers and sisters, husbands and wives, etc. If a commitment is a personal bond with the person to whom we have committed, and our intentions are honorable, why do we sometimes ignore the importance of keeping the commitment?

  Could this be an example of what the Bible instructs us in *Mark 4:38 "...The spirit is willing but the body is weak."*?

- Discuss and encourage the progress that some members of the group made with their commitment to heart-healthy living in Chapter 1 A Haughty Heart.

D) How would someone become committed to lifestyle changes while suffering with health problems? Do you think there would be a tendency to simply give up when they occur? Why or why not?

- Discuss how keeping our hearts receptive to His Word thwarts the devil's efforts to use illness and disease to prevent the seeds of doubt to be planted and rooted in our spirit. Focusing on God's strength helps us overcome our weaknesses and tendencies to give up in our efforts.

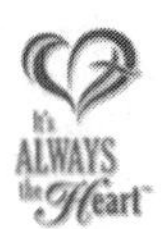

3. Personal Reflections: (25-30 minutes)

A) When it comes to resolving to live a healthier lifestyle, we often hear the resolution reduced to "will power". However, Jim Oliver knew that commitment was born from something stronger than simply his own "power". Think about your commitments, especially those that are difficult to achieve. Admit how your "will power" can not be enough and reveal how your *true power* can only come from God.

- Ask the group to honestly evaluate their motivations for losing weight and becoming healthier...is it born from the hope that they will be able to bask in the admiration of how others will see their accomplishments, for life changing benefits, or is Christ's glory the real motivation (or a combination of all motives)?

- Considering the Bible's stated lack of tolerance of pride and vanity in Proverbs, ask the group if it is ever o.k. for admiration of others to be a part of our lifestyle pursuits. (scripture references: Proverbs 11:2, Proverbs 16:18, Proverbs 23:29) It is also important to note that it is acceptable to be proud of our accomplishments as long as we turn over the glory to God for giving us the strength and guidance to succeed.

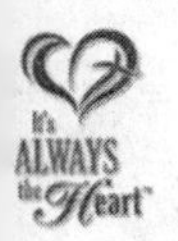

- Is *my* personal approach to committing to someone or something rooted in selflessness for Christ's glory?... or selfishness for personal glory? Elaborate on this reflection. Does it matter as long as the results are the same? Elaborate.

B) Jim Oliver invested his time and efforts into his wife, family and friends in order to "enjoy the fruits of his harvest and to have the type of relationship with God He desires". Do I invest in my friends and loved ones for the same reasons, or is it because it is society's expectation of me? What about *this group fellowship* - is my time investment by default because of society's expectations of what I should be doing or by design so I can grow spiritually and become closer with fellow brothers and sisters in Christ? Can it be some of both?

- Discuss the groups' response to these questions. However, in as much as the answers to these reflections may be significantly personal, please proceed sensitively.

- *Proverbs 18:24 (TNIV) One who has unreliable friends soon comes to ruin, but there is a friend who sticks closer than a brother.*

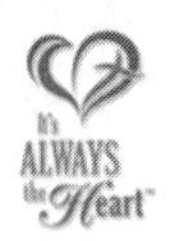

- *John 15: 12-13 My command is this: Love each other as I have loved you. Greater love has no one than this, that he lay down his life for his friends.*

- *Hebrews 10:24-25 (TNIV) And let us consider how we may spur one another on toward love and good deeds, not giving up meeting together, as some are in the habit of doing, but encouraging one another—and all the more as you see the Day approaching.*

C) If I encounter pain or resistance from something to which I've made a commitment - like patient Oliver's commitment to an exercise program – do I simply acknowledge it as something that "goes with the territory", or do I allow the painful encounter to diminish my resolve to seeing my commitment to a successful conclusion? How can I use God's Word to overcome the resistance I encounter to lifestyle changes?

- The primary focus here is to underscore the fundamental truth of Dr. Constantine's illustration in the Jim Oliver story... "*Yet the very essence of this story of Jim's transition to a stronger heart is not one of simply change...but, rather, the underlying commitment to change.*"

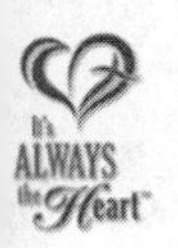

- Discuss the fact that all of us are prone to "giving up" in the face of adversity; but an unwavering relationship with God on a daily basis can strengthen our resolve.

- *2 Chronicles 16:9 For the eyes of the LORD range throughout the earth to strengthen those whose hearts are fully committed to him. …*

D) Jim Oliver was confident he would receive God's reward for good heart health "because of his offering his body to God." Considering my current state of physical health, can I truly say that I offer my body to God? Am I willing to commit to offering my heart and body to God? How do we deal with the fact that despite our best efforts, disease at times overcomes our physical bodies? Is this because we 'have done something wrong'? Elaborate on these questions.

- Discuss the Apostle Paul's clearly articulated position on presenting our bodies as a living sacrifice to God in *Romans 12:1-2 (TNIV) Therefore, I urge you, brothers and sisters, in view of God's mercy, to offer your bodies as a living sacrifice, holy and pleasing to God—this is true worship. Do not conform to the pattern of this world, but be transformed by the renewing of your mind. Then you will be able to test and approve what God's will is—his good, pleasing and perfect will.*

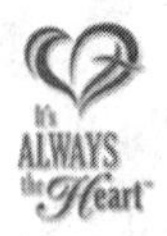

After reading this chapter, what has God revealed to my heart that will assist me in committing to the cultivation of a healthier physical and spiritual heart?

Chapter 5 Scripture Re-cap:

Psalm 37:5
Ephesians 6:12
Luke 6:45
Proverbs 3:2-3
Romans 12:2
Psalm 1:1-3 2

Romans 12:2
Psalm 1:1-3
Psalm 19:14
Romans 6:11-14
Philippians 4:6-7
Chronicles 16:9

Encourage group members to read and meditate on the scriptures referenced in each chapter.

Closing Prayer

NOTES

STUDY GUIDE

Small Group Participant Worksheet

Chapter 6

Faith Unaware

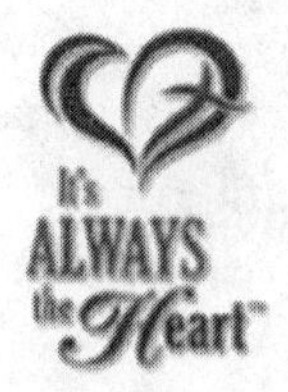

But without faith it is impossible to please Him, for he who comes to God must believe that He is, and that He is a rewarder of those who diligently seek Him.

Hebrews 11: 6 NKJV

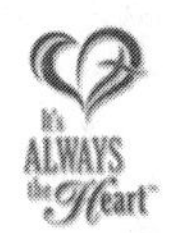

1. Preparation:

- Pray that God will use this message to strengthen the physical and spiritual hearts of you and all members in your group.
- Assign each meeting's opening prayer to a different group member.
- Read Chapter 6: Faith Unaware and become familiar with the scripture references in the chapter.
- Share your thoughts and reflections on the worksheet.
- Be sensitive to the fact that diet and exercise-related topics may sometimes cause personal embarrassment – particularly if a group member struggles with his/her diet and/or exercise commitment to the group. The group should maintain an "encouragement-only" environment regardless of a member's progress or lack thereof.
- Remember: the primary goal of each chapter is to illustrate and emphasize the importance of God's design of the inseparability of the physical and spiritual heart. Keep the discussion focused on the chapter's goal.
- Try to adhere to the time recommendations for each topic of group discussion.

2. Thoughts: (25-30 Minutes)

A) Leroy Harris is characterized as one who is 'unaware' of his role in life as a husband and child of God. He is also characterized as not knowing about that which he must do to care for his physical and spiritual heart. His days, weeks, years and life are ruled by the tasks related to his work which seem to define him. Claiming to be *unaware* would be somewhat difficult to defend in today's information-rich world. Once exposed to the truth, what does God say about knowing and not doing?

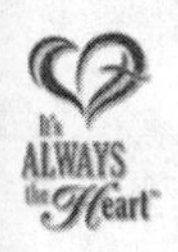

- The scriptures clearly identify the essence of our wrestling with *James 4:17* "knowing that which we are supposed to do… but not doing it". James summarizes the issue as it relates to our obedience to God's Word and commandments – and the consequence of not being obedient; *Anyone, then, who knows the good he ought to do and doesn't do it, sins.*

- *James 2:17* is also insightful on this topic: *In the same way, faith by itself, if it is not accompanied by action, is dead.*

B) Stop and think about those things we know we should or should not do but do not fulfill. Knowing what God says about hearers of the Word and doers of the Word, how do you think He feels about our disobedience? How does it make you feel when those close to you know but, nonetheless, refuse to do things important to us?

- Discussion of human disobedience often becomes relegated to a comparative example in the context of childlike disobedience. The Bible, however, provides a more adult-like approach by making it clear that when we are obedient we are yielding to God's authority and will. By contrast, when we are disobedient, we are yielding to our own will – and all the human frailties it represents.

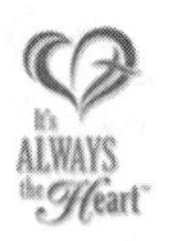

- *Deuteronomy 11:26-28 See, I am setting before you today a blessing and a curse— the blessing if you obey the commands of the LORD your God that I am giving you today; the curse if you disobey the commands of the LORD your God and turn from the way that I command you today by following other gods, which you have not known.*

- *1 Samuel 15: 22-23 But Samuel replied: "Does the LORD delight in burnt offerings and sacrifices as much as in obeying the LORD? To obey is better than sacrifice, and to heed is better than the fat of rams. For rebellion is like the sin of divination, and arrogance like the evil of idolatry. Because you have rejected the word of the LORD, he has rejected you as king."*

C) We are all occasionally guilty of using the "unaware" excuse as rationale to avoid focusing on our 'giants' – how does knowing what God says help us overcome these obstacles?

- In addition to the practical advice of obtaining the tools, information and other things we need to "slay the Goliaths" in our lives, Dr. Constantine reminds us in the telling of the Leroy Harris story that we must never give up by keeping the "eyes of our heart" opened to the eternal truth that everything is possible through Christ.

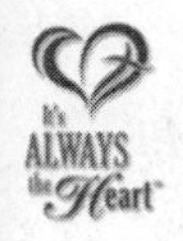

- *Ephesians 1:18 (TNIV) I pray that the eyes of your heart may be enlightened in order that you may know the hope to which he has called you, the riches of his glorious inheritance in his people,*

- *Mark 10:27 Jesus looked at them and said, "With man this is impossible, but not with God; all things are possible with God."*

D) Why do so many of us choose job, stress, illness or poor time management as an excuse to keep from doing the things we must for optimal heart health?

- Steer the discussion beyond the previously discussed obedience issue to one of laziness. Discuss the group's feelings about the applicability of the following scripture about excuses: *Ecclesiastes 11:4 (NKJV) He who observes the wind will not sow, And he who regards the clouds will not reap,* and *Proverbs 22:13 (NLT) The lazy person is full of excuses saying, "If I go outside, I might meet a lion in the street and be killed!"*

3. <u>Personal Reflections: (25-30 minutes)</u>

A) Do I live my life from day-to-day spiritually bankrupt with no time for God, or do I put Him first knowing that *what I do* for a living does not define who I am? Elaborate on how setting aside time for a relationship with the Lord impacts your day, your week, your job,… your life!

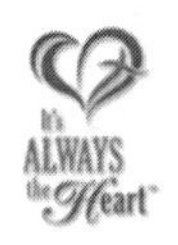

Scriptural reinforcement to the importance of making time for God in the midst of even the busiest of days when our hearts and minds are seemingly too full for even a simply prayer.

- *Ephesians 5:16 (NLT) Make the most of every opportunity for doing good in these evil days.*

- *Colossians 3:17 And whatever you do in word or deed, do all in the name of the Lord Jesus, giving thanks to God the Father through Him.*

- *Matthew 6:24 No one can serve two masters; for either he will hate the one and love the other, or else he will be loyal to the one and despise the other. You cannot serve God and mammon.*

B) Am I willing to commit to God, myself and the group to begin each day devoting time with God so I will no longer claim to be "unaware" of what He says about me? How will I make this part of my daily journey? Elaborate on why this is important.

Since a group member's approach to answering this question is consistent with the Chapter 1 question on commitment to spending time with God…suggest using it as a member's "look-back" at progress (or perhaps lack thereof)

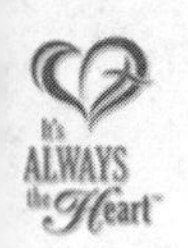

C) Do I live my life from day to day physically bankrupt with no time for caring for myself, or do I make it a priority to take care of my body…knowing my actions define who I am? What will I have to sacrifice to make sure I have time to eat right and exercise? How will it be worth it?

- An interesting exercise here entails asking the group to make a "High Priority" list (in rank order from most-to-least) of the most important daily occurrences in each member's life (or at least their perception of the most important). Then, upon completion, discuss the how many of the members actually prioritized taking care of their body.

D) Am I willing to commit to His Word, to understand His faithfulness and therefore become a more faithful child of God? Do I have a faithful heart, knowing that when I do what I am supposed to do, I will receive the outrageous promises of God, or do I have a wandering heart, not knowing what He says I can have? Elaborate on this reflection.

How can being faithful to the commitment of a healthier physical and spiritual heart impact my life?

- The primary definition of faithfulness means: *to adhere firmly and devotedly to a person, cause or idea…worthy of trust or belief.* The following scriptures define God's faithfulness and what it means to live as a faithful child of God:

- *Proverbs 28:20 A faithful man will be richly blessed, but one eager to get rich will not go unpunished.*

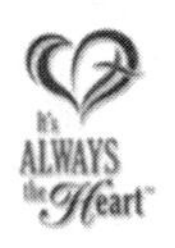

- *Luke 16: 10-12 (NKJV) "He who is faithful in what is least is faithful also in much; and he who is unjust in what is least is unjust also in much.*
- *Revelation 2:10 Do not be afraid of what you are about to suffer. I tell you, the devil will put some of you in prison to test you, and you will suffer persecution for ten days. Be faithful, even to the point of death, and I will give you the crown of life.*
- *James 1:22 Do not merely listen to the word, and so deceive yourselves. Do what it says.*

How is God trying to use this chapter to make my heart more aware of the need to prioritize as I travel along the highway of my life?

Chapter 6 Scripture Recap:

Hebrews 11:6
Luke 8:15
Psalm 18: 1-3
Matthew 11:28
Matthew 19:26
Hebrews 10: 35-36
James 1:5
Proverbs 3:13
Proverbs 4:7
Proverbs 8:11

Encourage group members to read and meditate on the scriptures referenced in each chapter.

Closing Prayer

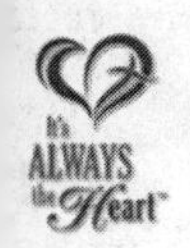

NOTES

STUDY GUIDE

Small Group Participant Worksheet

Chapter 7

Teaching Us To Trust

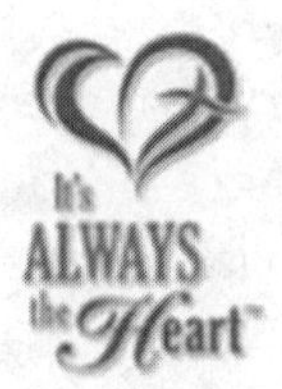

You will seek me and find me when you seek me with all your heart.

Jeremiah 29:13

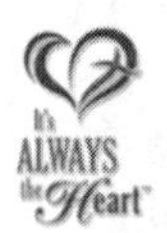

1. Preparation:

- Pray that God will use this message to strengthen the physical and spiritual hearts of you and all members in your group.
- Assign each meeting's opening prayer to a different group member.
- Read Chapter 7: Teaching Us To Trust and become familiar with the scripture references in the chapter.
- Share your thoughts and reflections on the worksheet.
- Be sensitive to the fact that diet and exercise-related topics may sometimes cause personal embarrassment – particularly if a group member struggles with his/her diet and/or exercise commitment to the group. The group should maintain an "encouragement-only" environment regardless of a member's progress or lack thereof.
- Remember: the primary goal of each chapter is to illustrate and emphasize the importance of God's design of the inseparability of the physical and spiritual heart. Keep the discussion focused on the chapter's goal.
- Try to adhere to the time recommendations for each topic of group discussion.

2. Thoughts: (25-30 Minutes)

A) Do you suppose prior to his heart attack, Pastor Jeremiah may have felt as though he was "shielded" from physical problems because God called him to teach His Word? Considering his line of work as a minister of the spiritual heart, do you suppose he might also have felt shielded from spiritual heart problems? Which of his heart problems do you think God felt needed the most attention? Why?

Think of the people around you (including yourself) with worldly power or influence – is there anything we do or have that really shields us from anything? Elaborate on this thought.

- If Pastor Jeremiah felt shielded from physical and spiritual heart problems because of his religious accomplishments, then he had unfortunately allowed self-righteousness to gain a foothold in his life. *Isaiah 64:6 (NKJV)* reminds us that *"But we are all like an unclean thing, And all our righteousnesses are like filthy rags;..."*

- It is Christ's righteousness in us that bears fruit in our pursuit of godly things…not our own feeble attempts. *2 Corinthians 5:21 God made him who had no sin to be sin for us, so that in him we might become the righteousness of God.*

- Discuss the significance of *Ephesians 6:10-17* – and each piece of God's armor described - as it relates to the only "real" shield anyone has against the devil's attacks. *Finally, be strong in the Lord and in his mighty power. Put on the full armor of God so that you can take your stand against the devil's schemes. For our struggle is not against flesh and blood, but against the rulers, against the authorities, against the powers of this dark world and against the spiritual forces of evil in the heavenly realms. Therefore put on the full armor of God, so that when the day of evil comes, you may be able to stand your ground,*

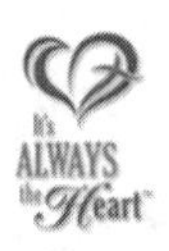

and after you have done everything, to stand. Stand firm then, with the belt of truth buckled around your waist, with the breastplate of righteousness in place, and with your feet fitted with the readiness that comes from the gospel of peace. In addition to all this, take up the shield of faith, with which you can extinguish all the flaming arrows of the evil one. Take the helmet of salvation and the sword of the Spirit, which is the word of God.

B) Are we as Christians ever guilty of using our faith as a "pass" for things that we are all guilty of – like the lack of exercise and/or our not seeking proper physical and spiritual nourishment? How else do we rationalize our behavior with our faith? What does God tell us about our faith without action on our part?

- In a non-judgmental manner, ask the group to list the ways they find themselves and other Christians rationalizing sinful behavior. As an example, one may illustrate the point with the fact that some people rationalize their overindulgence in alcohol as a much-needed "stress reliever". Another illustration one may highlight is the "entitlement mindset" that some Christians exhibit when they choose to forego exercise in order to indulge in the rest and relaxation they "deserve" after a hard day's work.

C) It is easy to tell someone to trust God to lead us through a trial when we are not facing the problem ourselves. How do we act when a trial comes our way? Do you think we have more

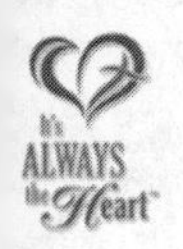

credibility and are better witnesses when we have actually gone through things ourselves? Do you think this could be part of God's *master plan* to use those who have successfully gone through trials as visible examples of His healing powers in our lives?

How do our trials allow us to give a more credible testimony regarding how God's truth came to life during our struggle?

- Most of us react to trials in our lives in varying ways. Feelings of anger, bitterness, frustration, revenge, depression, unfair treatment and even denial are all common reactions to our trials – whether self-inflicted or not. However, God has provided us with the perfect example of how best to react through the account of Jesus' sufferings – with peacefulness and patience.

- The following scripture gives us a balanced view of trials-as-discipline that reassures us of God in our lives: *Hebrews 12: 5-7 And you have forgotten that word of encouragement that addresses you as sons:"My son, do not make light of the Lord's discipline, and do not lose heart when he rebukes you, because the Lord disciplines those he loves, and he punishes everyone he accepts as a son." Endure hardship as discipline; God is treating you as sons. For what son is not disciplined by his father?*

- While it may be difficult to accept on surface, embracing our trials is the essence of this often quoted verse in *James (1:2) Consider it pure joy, my brothers, whenever you face trials of many kinds.*

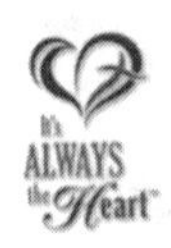

D) Is it simply "human nature", or is there some other reason(s) why we so easily dismiss lifestyle behavior that we know to be detrimental to our physical and spiritual health? Elaborate on this and identify the other reason(s) we behave in this manner.

- As discussed in other chapters, there are many reasons (most of which are simply excuses) why we quickly dismiss lifestyle behavior. However, whether or not they are "human nature" is really not worthy of pondering. God's Word makes our sinful nature crystal clear by showing us that we often find ourselves resisting to the submission to the Lordship and authority of Christ. *Ephesians 2:10 For we are God's workmanship, created in Christ Jesus to do good works, which God prepared in advance for us to do.*

3. Personal Reflections: (25-30 minutes)

A) When I truly examine my attitude about diet and exercise, do I – as Pastor Jeremiah – simply tell myself that the demands of my job, family, etc. prevent me from eating right and exercising? What can I do to overcome these excuses and become more committed to a healthier lifestyle?

- It may be encouraging (and eye opening) to ask someone in the group who has overcome their rationalizing of diet and exercise issues to share the secrets of their success and progress toward better physical health with the group. How am I open to trying a plan that has worked for someone else even if it takes me out of my comfort zone?

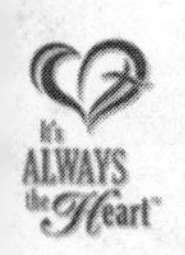

B) What about my spiritual heart health, do I use the same "too" excuses – too busy, too tired, too early, too late, too much, etc. - to prevent me from daily heart nourishment which only the scriptures can provide? How can I get beyond the excuses?

- Often, our apathy toward daily spiritual practice lies in a simple lack of enthusiasm. Use the following scripture as the benchmark of maintaining a positive, optimistic attitude of zeal for daily heart nourishment:

- *Galatians 6:9 Let us not become weary in doing good, for at the proper time we will reap a harvest if we do not give up.*

- *Romans 12:11 Never be lacking in zeal, but keep your spiritual fervor, serving the Lord.*

- *Philippians 3:12-14 Not that I have already obtained all this, or have already been made perfect, but I press on to take hold of that for which Christ Jesus took hold of me. Brothers, I do not consider myself yet to have taken hold of it. But one thing I do: Forgetting what is behind and straining toward what is ahead, I press on toward the goal to win the prize for which God has called me heavenward in Christ Jesus.*

- *Deuteronomy 17:19 It is to be with him, and he is to read it all the days of his life so that he may learn to revere the* LORD *his God and follow carefully all the words of this law and these decrees*

C) No matter who we are or what our experience, we all need to seek godly counsel for ourselves in times of need. Do we seek

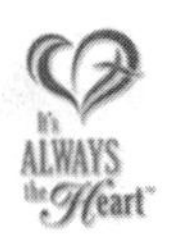

Him when things are going well… "Oh God, we praise and worship You" and forget about Him when distracted by illness/ trials? Or do we forget about Him when things are going well, only to turn to Him at a time of need, asking Him "Oh God, where are You now?" as we plead for a solution to our dilemma? Elaborate on this reflection. How should our relationship with God look?

- The personal reflections to these questions will likely vary among group members. However, *Philippians 4: 11-12* provides meaningful scriptural insight and valuable instruction as to how to live a life in Christ through the experiences of both good and bad times: *I am not saying this because I am in need, for I have learned to be content whatever the circumstances. I know what it is to be in need, and I know what it is to have plenty. I have learned the secret of being content in any and every situation, whether well fed or hungry, whether living in plenty or in want.*

D) Should we not go through trials standing in faith, trusting in God's infinite wisdom as we battle in His strength? How do you think God wants our hearts and focus on Him daily?

- Teaching Us To Trust shows us how to withstand our trials by standing in faith, trusting God's infinite wisdom, and by waging our battle through trials and tribulations armed with His strength. When it comes to physical and spiritual heart health, the daily requirement is a focus on the intake of the Word of God as much as on our intake of daily physical nourishment.

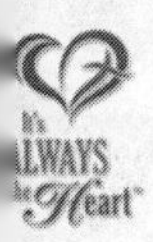

How can I use the core lesson of trusting in God embodied in this chapter to begin a journey, ***today,*** towards a destination of better physical and spiritual heart health?

Chapter 7 Scripture Recap:

Jeremiah 29:13
Isaiah 53:5
Psalm 37:5
1 Corinthians 6:19-20
Jeremiah 30:17
1 Corinthians 9:24-25
Philippians 4:13
James 1:2-4
Romans 8:28

Encourage group members to read and meditate on the scriptures referenced in each chapter.

Closing Prayer

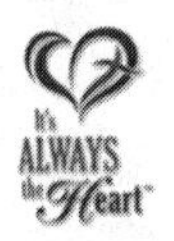

NOTES

STUDY GUIDE

Small Group Participant Worksheet

Chapter 8

Living In Denial

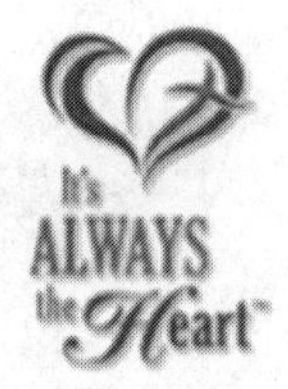

If we endure, We shall also reign with Him. If we deny Him, He also will deny us.

2 Timothy 2: 12(NKJV)

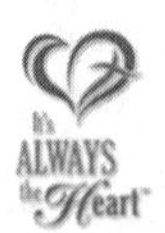

1. Preparation:

- Pray that God will use this message to strengthen the physical and spiritual hearts of you and all members in your group.
- Assign each meeting's opening prayer to a different group member.
- Read Chapter 8: Living In Denial and become familiar with the scripture references in the chapter.
- Share your thoughts and reflections on the worksheet.
- Be sensitive to the fact that diet and exercise-related topics may sometimes cause personal embarrassment – particularly if a group member struggles with his/her diet and/or exercise commitment to the group. The group should maintain an "encouragement-only" environment regardless of a member's progress or lack thereof.
- Remember: the primary goal of each chapter is to illustrate and emphasize the importance of God's design of the inseparability of the physical and spiritual heart. Keep the discussion focused on the chapter's goal.
- Try to adhere to the time recommendations for each topic of group discussion.

2. Thoughts: (25-30 Minutes)

A) If, as Dr. Constantine suggests early in the chapter that "…we are all often only inches away from the threshold of life to death – all day, everyday…" why do we not spend time thinking about that inescapable fact? Is it a statement of complete confidence in our salvation, denial, or simply a subject that represents too much fear for us to wrap our minds around?

- Often the denial of our mortality is rooted in fear…the fear of when and how we will die. As devoted followers

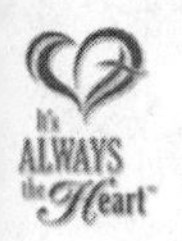

of God, we should abandon the futile efforts to deny death and accept the fact that the death of our earthly bodies is simply an inescapable part of God's plan for eternal life for all who place their hope in Him. Paul provides a hopeful attitude toward death in *Philippians 1:21-24 For to me, to live is Christ and to die is gain. If I am to go on living in the body, this will mean fruitful labor for me. Yet what shall I choose? I do not know! I am torn between the two: I desire to depart and be with Christ, which is better by far; but it is more necessary for you that I remain in the body.*

- Regarding *when* we die, the scriptures clearly inform us that no one knows; and that we must always be prepared: *Luke 12: 39-40 But understand this: If the owner of the house had known at what hour the thief was coming, he would not have let his house be broken into. You also must be ready, because the Son of Man will come at an hour when you do not expect him."* How does this scripture affect you? Does it encourage you? Discourage you? Frighten you? Why?

B) Do you have family or friends who have faced a life or death event and lived to tell about it? What was the effect the event had on the manner in which they led their lives after the event? How did this change the manner in which you live?

- In light of the fact that each group member will have a different description of post-event effects on friends or

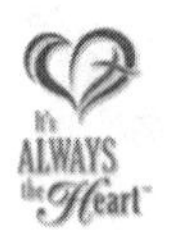

family raised by this question - encourage them to find supportive scripture to illustrate the manner in which the friend or family member should have lived life after the life-threatening event.

- Resolve the discussion with *2 Corinthians 5:8*, which reflects that which should be every Christian's attitude regarding death- whether pre or post a life-threatening event: *We are confident, I say, and would prefer to be away from the body and at home with the Lord.*

C) The main character, Jean Watson, was a professing Christian, but admitted that she rarely "turned to Him on a daily basis". How many of us only turn to Him occasionally in a time of need? Why not daily?

- Staying in daily fellowship with God requires devotion and practice. The following scriptures convict us of our need to walk daily with Him:

- *1 John 1:6 If we claim to have fellowship with him yet walk in the darkness, we lie and do not live by the truth.*

- *Philippians 3:12 Not that I have already obtained all this, or have already been made perfect, but I press on to take hold of that for which Christ Jesus took hold of me.*

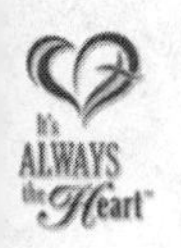

- Ask yourself how you think God desires us to fellowship with Him, and, if anyone can expect to mature in their Christianity with only occasional fellowship with Him.

D) Denial of the need for exercise, a proper diet, to stop smoking, to avoid overeating, and countless other lifestyle issues are at the root of physical heart problems. Likewise, is denial of the need for a daily relationship with Christ at the root of our spiritual problems, or is it something even more important? How can a stronger relationship with God help strengthen our resolve to take better care of ourselves physically and emotionally? How are you willing to put down this cloak of denial and accept the opportunity of a daily relationship with Jesus Christ that He offers you?

- Pleasing God by taking care of our physical and spiritual hearts is an act of worship, and – among other Christ-honoring things – a statement of our thankfulness for the faithfulness of His countless blessings. *Romans 12:1 Therefore, I urge you, brothers, in view of God's mercy, to offer your bodies as living sacrifices, holy and pleasing to God—this is your spiritual act of worship.*

3. <u>Personal Reflections: (25-30 minutes)</u>

A) Am I aware of the binding between my physical and spiritual heart, or, like so many believers, do I deny that there is a coupling or intertwining and treat the two separately?

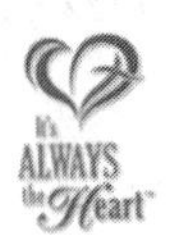

- The description of Jesus' life in the book of Luke is the perfect example of how we are to live a complete physical and spiritual life: *Luke 2:52 And Jesus grew in wisdom and stature, and in favor with God and men.* In essence, this verse tells us that Jesus grew both physically and spiritually – together, not separately – relative to God the Father and the society around him.

B) Do I understand that neglect of my physical heart can cost me my life here on earth…and that neglect of my spiritual heart can cost me my eternal life? Describe how this question resonates with you. Ultimately is one type of neglect of heart worse than the other? Why or why not?

- *1 Timothy 4:8 (NKJV) For bodily exercise profits a little, but godliness is profitable for all things, having promise of the life that now is and of that which is to come.*

C) When we become motivated to make beneficial life changes, why do you think it is hard to make lasting change? If it is common sense to eat healthier and exercise daily, why do we need the support of biblical principles to maintain these lifestyle changes? How do biblical principles make it easier for lifestyle changes to become permanent?

- It is our prideful nature to think that we can do things without the on-going nurture and support of God's Word. To prevent falling back into a neglectful pattern of living, we must maintain a humble attitude

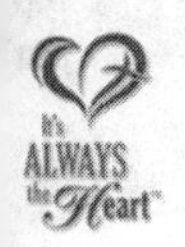

of submission to His instruction and encouragement in order to remind ourselves daily of both the earthly and heavenly importance of physical and spiritual nourishment and exercise. *1 Corinthians 10:12 So, if you think you are standing firm, be careful that you don't fall!*

D) What role do you feel the devil has, if any, in derailing us from our attempts to make a lasting change toward taking better care of our physical and spiritual hearts?

- This may be a good time for an open discussion among group members regarding the concept of the devil and why or why not various members believe the way they do regarding this subject.

- Supportive Scripture:

- *James 4:7 Submit yourselves, then, to God. Resist the devil, and he will flee from you.*

- *Matthew 4:10 Jesus said to him, "Away from me, Satan! For it is written: 'Worship the Lord your God, and serve him only."*

- *2 Corinthians 2:11 in order that Satan might not outwit us. For we are not unaware of his schemes.*

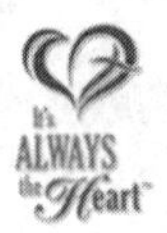

How can I use what I've learned in this chapter and use it to drive denial out of my heart, mind and spirit?

Chapter 8 Scripture Recap
2 Timothy 2:12
Proverbs 3:5-6
Jeremiah 18:1-6
Exodus 14:14
Hebrews 12: 12-13
2 Timothy 4:7
Philippians 4:7
Psalm 55:22

Encourage group members to read and meditate on the scriptures referenced in each chapter.

Closing Prayer

NOTES

STUDY GUIDE

Small Group Participant Worksheet

Chapter 9

Living In Fear of Dying

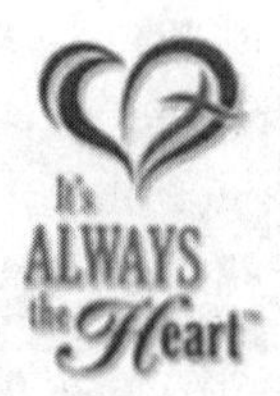

Keep your heart with all diligence, For out of it spring the issues of life.

Proverbs 4:23 (NKJV)

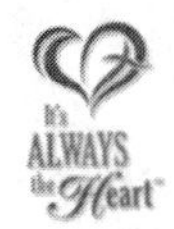

1. Preparation:

- Pray that God will use this message to strengthen the physical and spiritual hearts of you and all members in your group.
- Assign each meeting's opening prayer to a different group member.
- Read Chapter 9: Living In Fear of Dying and become familiar with the scripture references in the chapter.
- Share your thoughts and reflections on the worksheet.
- Be sensitive to the fact that diet and exercise-related topics may sometimes cause personal embarrassment – particularly if a group member struggles with his/her diet and/or exercise commitment to the group. The group should maintain an "encouragement-only" environment regardless of a member's progress or lack thereof.
- Remember: the primary goal of each chapter is to illustrate and emphasize the importance of God's design of the inseparability of the physical and spiritual heart. Keep the discussion focused on the chapter's goal.
- Try to adhere to the time recommendations for each topic of group discussion.

2. Thoughts: (25-30 Minutes)

A) Almost everyone is guilty at one time or another of – even if only for a day or two – allowing fear to rule, if not ruin, their hearts and minds. How do the scriptures instruct us to shake off the fear when we sometimes find ourselves in its grasp?

- Although many people are reluctant to openly discuss their fears (perhaps in an attempt to hide a personal weakness), ask one of the "braver" spirits in the group (or if self study – you) to name their greatest fear, and how they have (or are attempting to) overcome it.

- Scripture assurances for helping us deal with fear:

- *Isaiah 35:4 say to those with fearful hearts, "Be strong, do not fear; your God will come, he will come with vengeance; with divine retribution he will come to save you."*

- *Psalm 23:4 Even though I walk through the valley of the shadow of death, I will fear no evil, for you are with me; your rod and your staff, they comfort me.*

- *Deuteronomy 31:6 Be strong and courageous. Do not be afraid or terrified because of them, for the LORD your God goes with you; he will never leave you nor forsake you."*

B) As the character, Jim, found himself convinced by the devil that he was in a hopeless situation, his fears worsened and "…the reality, presence and purpose of Christ was not there". Stop and think of the last time you were gripped by fear…did you also feel as though Christ was nowhere to be found? What light did the Apostle Paul shed on hopelessness?

- The Apostle Paul faced countless fear-filled moments – from menacing enemies to storms on the high seas. However, he shows us that finding hope in the midst of hopelessness lies in our understanding that our circumstances are not random occurrences without purpose and meaning.

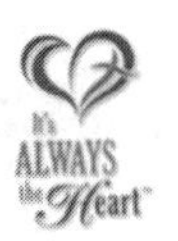

- *Romans 5:3-5 Not only so, but we also rejoice in our sufferings, because we know that suffering produces perseverance; perseverance, character; and character, hope. And hope does not disappoint us, because God has poured out his love into our hearts by the Holy Spirit, whom he has given us.*

- *Isaiah 41:10 So do not fear, for I am with you; do not be dismayed, for I am your God. I will strengthen you and help you; I will uphold you with my righteous right hand.*

C) Dr. Constantine reminds us in this chapter that the human heart beats, on average, over 100,000 times per day…yet we often go days, weeks, months, years, or even a lifetime without acknowledging its importance to our very existence here on earth. How is our indifference to its importance the same or similar to our frequent indifference to the heart's importance in maintaining a healthy relationship with our Creator of this most marvelous life-giving organ?

- Half-hearted (no pun intended) attempts to nurture a relationship with our Creator are often symptoms of our human indifference and lack of appreciation for His blessings in our lives. This same indifference is sometimes present in our attitudes toward leading a healthier physical and spiritual lifestyle. Fervently seeking and maintaining a strong relationship with our Father is the most important pursuit we as believers can undertake.

- Scripture Support for seeking and maintaining a healthy relationship with God:

- *Jeremiah 29:13 You will seek me and find me when you seek me with all your heart*

- *Psalm 19:14 May the words of my mouth and the meditation of my heart be pleasing in your sight, O LORD, my Rock and my Redeemer.*

- *Isaiah 29:13-15 The Lord says: "These people come near to me with their mouth and honor me with their lips, but their hearts are far from me. Their worship of me is made up only of rules taught by men. Therefore once more I will astound these people with wonder upon wonder; the wisdom of the wise will perish, the intelligence of the intelligent will vanish." Woe to those who go to great depths to hide their plans from the LORD, who do their work in darkness and think, "Who sees us? Who will know?"*

D) As testing confirmed, it was not Jim's physical heart as the cause of his symptoms. How was Jim's desire for things in life in which he was not willing to put forth the effort, an example of how the heart is always at the root of the problem?

- Ask group members to share their thoughts about how the heart is always at the root of personal problems.

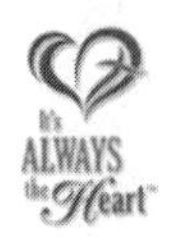

- Resolve the discussion with these excerpts from Wiersbe's Expository Commentary about guarding our hearts: "Guard your heart above anything else you have because it determines the kind of life you will live. The heart is the "master-control" of our life; a wrong heart produces a wrong life. To allow sin into the heart is to pollute the entire life."

- No matter how much we safe-keep our material possessions or protect our body from personal illness or injury, our failure to *ensure* the safe-keeping of our all-important hearts, will affect all areas of life.

3. <u>Personal Reflections: (25-30 minutes)</u>

A) Do I willingly open my heart and mind to God to take away fears that cripple my Christian walk, or do I allow the devil to keep them harbored in the forefront of my thinking? How can my relationship with Father God overcome these fears that can consume my heart and mind?

- Fear can often be viewed as faith in the devil that allows him free passage into our lives: *Job 3:25 What I feared has come upon me; what I dreaded has happened to me.*

- Comfort in the face of fear:

- *Psalm 62:8 Trust in him at all times, O people; pour out your hearts to him, for God is our refuge.*

- *Romans 6:6 For we know that our old self was crucified with him so that the body of sin might be done away with, that we should no longer be slaves to sin—*

- *Matthew 6:34 Therefore do not worry about tomorrow, for tomorrow will worry about itself. Each day has enough trouble of it's own.*

B) Am I willing to submit to a commitment to cultivate a healthy physical and spiritual heart, so that I may find myself in the caress of His grace rather than the grips of my fear? What must I do to solidify this commitment?

- In conjunction with the "fear" discussion, this may be a timely group moment to "look-back" at the progress made by those who made the commitment to begin leading a healthier lifestyle in Chapter 1 A Haughty Heart. (Remember, these should be encouraging-only discussions so as not to promote embarrassment toward someone who has perhaps not been diligent in keeping their earlier healthy lifestyle commitment.)

C) Do we claim disease as "my heart problem, my cholesterol problem, my cancer, etc…" or feel predestined for a disease because of "my family history" or, because "it runs in my family" and take ownership of these diseases as if we have no control over our lives? Or do we turn to God's Word for the solution to rid these things from our lives – which frees us from the bondage disease has in our life? Elaborate.

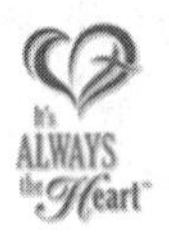

- Sometimes we choose to "own" our problems and diseases almost as if to confirm our identities. However, Christ is our hope and constantly intercedes to the Father on our behalf to help us remove the bondage of disease to establish our true identity in Him.

- *Romans 8:34 Who is he that condemns? Christ Jesus, who died—more than that, who was raised to life—is at the right hand of God and is also interceding for us.*

- *Matthew 9:35(TNIV) Jesus went through all the towns and villages, teaching in their synagogues, proclaiming the good news of the kingdom and healing every disease and sickness.*

D) How can I promise myself and those in my fellowship that I will put aside the time-worn excuses that prevent me from enjoying the fullness of Christ?

- *2 Corinthians 12: 9-10 But he said to me, "My grace is sufficient for you, for my power is made perfect in weakness." Therefore I will boast all the more gladly about my weaknesses, so that Christ's power may rest on me. That is why, for Christ's sake, I delight in weaknesses, in insults, in hardships, in persecutions, in difficulties. For when I am weak, then I am strong.*

How can I use what I have learned in this chapter to stand confidently, overcoming the baseless fear in my life?

Chapter 9 Scripture Recap:
Proverbs 4:23
Colossians 3:23
Proverbs 4:20-23
1 Corinthians 3:6
James 4:8
Hebrews 12:11

Encourage group members to read and meditate on the scriptures referenced in each chapter.

Closing Prayer

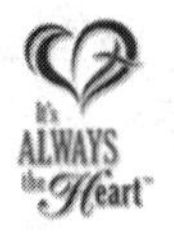

NOTES

Chapter 10

When Is It Over

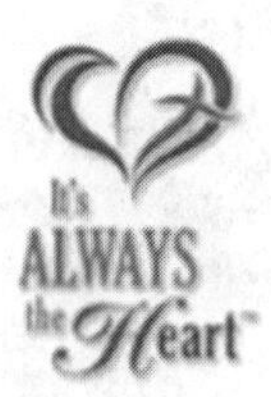

It is better to go to a house of mourning than to go to a house of feasting, for death is the destiny of every man; the living should take this to heart.

Ecclesiastes 7:2

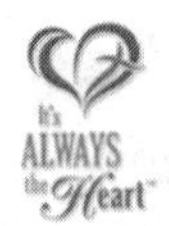

1. Preparation:

- Pray that God will use this message to strengthen the physical and spiritual hearts of you and all members in your group.
- Assign each meeting's opening prayer to a different group member.
- Read Chapter 10: When Is It Over and become familiar with the scripture references in the chapter.
- Share your thoughts and reflections on the worksheet.
- Be sensitive to the fact that diet and exercise-related topics may sometimes cause personal embarrassment – particularly if a group member struggles with his/her diet and/or exercise commitment to the group. The group should maintain an "encouragement-only" environment regardless of a member's progress or lack thereof.
- Remember: the primary goal of each chapter is to illustrate and emphasize the importance of God's design of the inseparability of the physical and spiritual heart. Keep the discussion focused on the chapter's goal.
- Try to adhere to the time recommendations for each topic of group discussion.

2. Thoughts: (25-30 Minutes)

A) As discussed in the previous chapter, most of us avoid thinking or talking about death at all costs…yet it is something we will all face – some sooner than others. Is our avoidance of the inevitable based in fear of our earthly absence, God's judgment upon our lives, or is it simply human procrastination towards our having to face the reality of death?

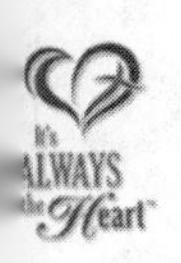

Where does Dr. Constantine point us to reassurance in the scriptures of how we must mentally approach the end to our earthly lives? Are we fearful of the unseen but 'known' promise of God, finding it hard to get our mind around the fact that it is really not over when it is over?

- Perhaps the best starting place for this discussion is to point to a definitive resolution of death itself from a scriptural perspective:

- *2 Timothy 1: 9-10 who has saved us and called us to a holy life—not because of anything we have done but because of his own purpose and grace. This grace was given us in Christ Jesus before the beginning of time, but it has now been revealed through the appearing of our Savior, Christ Jesus, who has destroyed death and has brought life and immortality to light through the gospel.*

- The group should be encouraged to read and meditate on the entire chapter 15 of first Corinthians which provides a comprehensive summation on death, and why we should not overtly harbor fears of it:

- *1 Corinthians 15: 56-57 The sting of death is sin, and the power of sin is the law. But thanks be to God! He gives us the victory through our Lord Jesus Christ.*

B) Taking the above thought a step further…In spite of her age and underlying medical issues that had resulted in her gradual mental and physical decline, it is pointed out in the chapter that Mrs. Whitt "...had not spent much time thinking about the end of her life." How can an older adult suffering from multiple life-threatening medical issues – and the family for that matter - simply ignore their own mortality?

- It has been said that fear of death is "hard-wired" into our bodies as it was not a part of God's original plan, but a necessary response to evil and sin in the world. Thus it may be impractical to think that we can simply altogether avoid thinking about the end of our lives. Certain scriptures, however, should give rise to comforting us in our fear of the unknown surrounding death: *Philippians 3:20-21 But our citizenship is in heaven. And we eagerly await a Savior from there, the Lord Jesus Christ, who, by the power that enables him to bring everything under his control, will transform our lowly bodies so that they will be like his glorious body. 1 Corinthians 6:14 By his power God raised the Lord from the dead, and he will raise us also*

C) It appeared that Mrs. Whitt's family's primary concern was to ensure her wishes of "...not being kept alive on a ventilator" were honored. Is it possible that we are all so fixated upon the alleviation of human pain and suffering that focus on a loved one's "final moments" are misprioritized? Beyond the prevention of physical suffering, what are the most important priorities a family should address if faced with a loved one's final moments?

- The importance of salvation as told in the story of the rich man and Lazarus is an appropriate parallel to the

question of important priorities when facing the final moments of life. Ask someone in the group to read Luke 16: 19-31 and discuss the group's observations on the message God is sending us in this story.

- *"There was a rich man who was dressed in purple and fine linen and lived in luxury every day. At his gate was laid a beggar named Lazarus, covered with sores and longing to eat what fell from the rich man's table. Even the dogs came and licked his sores. "The time came when the beggar died and the angels carried him to Abraham's side. The rich man also died and was buried. In hell, where he was in torment, he looked up and saw Abraham far away, with Lazarus by his side. So he called to him, 'Father Abraham, have pity on me and send Lazarus to dip the tip of his finger in water and cool my tongue, because I am in agony in this fire.' "But Abraham replied, 'Son, remember that in your lifetime you received your good things, while Lazarus received bad things, but now he is comforted here and you are in agony. And besides all this, between us and you a great chasm has been fixed, so that those who want to go from here to you cannot, nor can anyone cross over from there to us. "He answered, 'Then I beg you, father, send Lazarus to my father's house, for I have five brothers. Let him warn them, so that they will not also come to this place of torment.' "Abraham replied, 'They have Moses and the Prophets; let them listen to them.' "'No, father Abraham,' he said, 'but if someone from the dead goes to them, they will repent.' "He said to him, 'If they do not listen to Moses and the Prophets, they will not be convinced even if someone rises from the dead.'"*

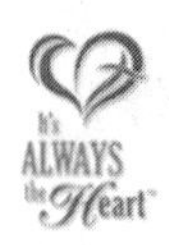

D) A funeral has been called a "celebration of life". If we are reassured by that which God tells us about the death of those of us who accept Jesus as Lord, why are we so sad and tearful when our loved ones pass away after a long and fruitful life?

- Admittedly, there are a myriad of saddening thoughts in the face of "celebrating" someone's life-after-death… personal loss, fear of our own mortality, etc. The concept of life everlasting in Heaven – surrounded with all of a family's loved ones – is also difficult when standing before a friend or loved one's lifeless body. *1 John 3:1-3* gives us assurance in the midst of our emotional uncertainty that the afterlife is a certainty: *How great is the love the Father has lavished on us, that we should be called children of God! And that is what we are! The reason the world does not know us is that it did not know him. Dear friends, now we are children of God, and what we will be has not yet been made known. But we know that when he appears, we shall be like him, for we shall see him as he is. Everyone who has this hope in him purifies himself, just as he is pure.*

3. Personal Reflections: (25-30 minutes)

A) If faced with a life & death moment like Mrs. Whitt's with family surrounding me, what do I want them to say to the medical staff attending me? Would their statements be guided by the condition of my physical *and* spiritual heart? In a situation like Mrs. Whitt, would it be reasonable to proceed with an emergency cardiac procedure to "squeeze out" more time on earth; or, would I prefer to go peacefully knowing my place in Heaven is secure?

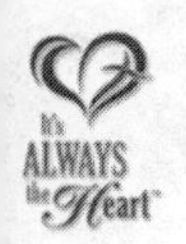

- Perhaps the primary reason to aggressively attempt to give a patient more time on earth, would focus on their need to accept Christ as Savior. Members of the group however, will likely list and be willing to discuss other reasons for life-saving measures.

- *1 John 2:25 And this is what he promised us—even eternal life.*

B) In the middle of my doubts and fears, how can I take to heart that which Dr. Constantine reminds us of in the chapter when he says "… God is always our comforter…there is never a time even during death when we are alone." ?

- All of us occasionally find ourselves conflicted between our humanly doubts and the promises of eternal life. To overcome it, God has provided us His Holy Word to help eliminate our doubts and fears:

- *Hebrews 6:10-12 God is not unjust; he will not forget your work and the love you have shown him as you have helped his people and continue to help them. We want each of you to show this same diligence to the very end, in order to make your hope sure. We do not want you to become lazy, but to imitate those who through faith and patience inherit what has been promised.*

- *2 Timothy 1:9-10 who has saved us and called us to a holy life—not because of anything we have done but because*

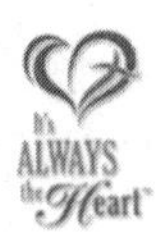

of his own purpose and grace. This grace was given us in Christ Jesus before the beginning of time, but it has now been revealed through the appearing of our Savior, Christ Jesus, who has destroyed death and has brought life and immortality to light through the gospel.

- *Revelation 21:3-4 And I heard a loud voice from the throne saying, "Now the dwelling of God is with men, and he will live with them. They will be his people, and God himself will be with them and be their God. He will wipe every tear from their eyes. There will be no more death or mourning or crying or pain, for the old order of things has passed away."*

C) I admit that I rarely give death a second thought and, therefore, why must I search God's Word as the first step in understanding that a day-to-day relationship with Christ is the foundation upon which I can embrace my inevitable departure from my earthly body for Heaven? How will this help me live in peace at a time when my earthly life is coming to an end?

- *Romans 5:12-21* clearly explains the essence of Christian belief of death through Adam and life through Christ: *Therefore, just as sin entered the world through one man, and death through sin, and in this way death came to all men, because all sinned— for before the law was given, sin was in the world. But sin is not taken into account when there is no law. Nevertheless, death reigned from the time of Adam to the time of Moses, even over those who did not sin by breaking a command, as did Adam, who was a pattern of the one to come. But the gift is not like the trespass. For if the many died by the trespass of the one man, how much more did God's grace and the*

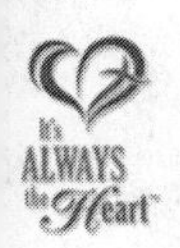

gift that came by the grace of the one man, Jesus Christ, overflow to the many! Again, the gift of God is not like the result of the one man's sin: The judgment followed one sin and brought condemnation, but the gift followed many trespasses and brought justification. For if, by the trespass of the one man, death reigned through that one man, how much more will those who receive God's abundant provision of grace and of the gift of righteousness reign in life through the one man, Jesus Christ. Consequently, just as the result of one trespass was condemnation for all men, so also the result of one act of righteousness was justification that brings life for all men. For just as through the disobedience of the one man the many were made sinners, so also through the obedience of the one man the many will be made righteous. The law was added so that the trespass might increase. But where sin increased, grace increased all the more, so that, just as sin reigned in death, so also grace might reign through righteousness to bring eternal life through Jesus Christ our Lord.

D) It is a well known fact that we use the majority of our lifetime health care expense in the last 5 years of life. Without getting morbid and mapping out our death, funeral and obituary, at a certain age, like Mrs. Whitt, how would it be reasonable to have a plan for that time so it will not come as a surprise and cause panic when faced with life threatening circumstances?

- With a generous measure of sensitivity in tow, it may be interesting (and perhaps even motivating to others) to hear from group members willing to share their attempts at end-of-life planning.

- *Psalm 89:48 What man can live and not see death, or save himself from the power of the grave? "Selah"*

How has this chapter influenced your thinking about the approach to understanding and accepting the scriptural fact that everyone has a date with death?

Chapter 10 Scripture Re-cap:

Ecclesiastes 7:2
John 5:24
Ephesians 2:8-9
Matthew 6:34
Isaiah 57:1-2
John 11:25-26
Hebrews 9:27
Isaiah 53:12
John 3:16
2 Corinthians 5:8
Psalm 119:112
Hebrews 4:12-13

Encourage group members to read and meditate on the scriptures referenced in each chapter.

Closing Prayer

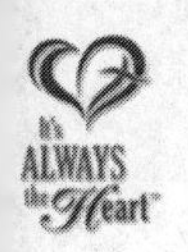

NOTES